The Complete Dr. Sebi Cookbook

Discover How To Detox, Cleanse, and Revitalize Your Body with Alkaline Diet. Find Out the Dr. Sebi Food List and Products and Cook Mouthwatering Meals

Sophia Parks

Table of contents

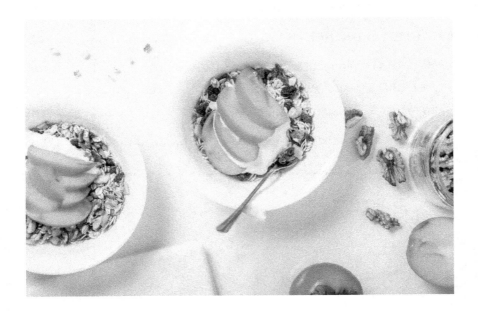

Introduction

Dr. Sebi is a well-known pathologist, naturalist, biochemist and herbalist. He visited different areas from Central and South America, Africa, North America, and the Caribbean. He made a lot of research and personally experienced several herbs; based on his research, he developed a specific approach and deduced technique for curing different diseases affecting the human body by using herbs deeply rooted in more than 30 years of practice.

His plans include a quite stringent dietary routine and costly supplements, which promises to detoxify the human body and prevent it from different diseases and restore alkalinity in the body. Dr. Sebi claims that His Diet plans can greatly help fight against several common diseases, including High blood pressure, diabetes, obesity, liver disorder, kidney problems and many others, which will be discussed in upcoming chapters.

Chapter 1. Dr. Sebi Diet

Alkaline foods are considered some of the healthiest foods that exist on earth. These are highly recommended to those suffering from chronic diseases because of a compromised immune system, low energy, anxiety, and headaches. On top of the list red meat, pasta, candies, and dairy products are those foods which cause acid in the body are typically consumed more than other products. It's not an easy task to change someone's diet, especially in those cases when it's supposed to be a sudden or dramatic change. You need to find a solution and ways to agree with someone to change his/her routine to lower the acid load in the body and follow healthy habits regarding eating routines and diet plans to enhance health. There are many dieting debates between the latest diet documentaries and other influencers promoting their current favorite diet pills. With lots of contradictory facts about which food and diet are better, even if it is advocated by somebody who seems credible, it is difficult to differentiate reality from fiction. For example, take Sebi's Diet, which is also 2019 's second most-searched diet on Google. Many might assume that this is a physician's created software. It is also assumed that Alfredo Bowman, the founder, was a herbalist, not a medical doctor. Dr. Sebi Diet is highly restrictive in nature, with a lack of protein intake and some vitamins. It mainly focuses on consuming a plant-based diet and avoid refined foods. Dr. Sebi believed that most diseases are caused by mucus and an increased amount of acidity in the body. He argued that by using an alkaline-based food, diseases could not occur.

1.1 What is the alkaline diet of Doctor Sebi?

A famous plant-based diet plan has been formulated by late Dr. Sebi, known by his name the Sebi's diet, also known as a Sebi's alkaline diet. This diet helps by removing toxic waste in the body by alkalizing the blood. It is believed that this process revitalizes your cells. The diet normally depends, along with several supplements, on consuming a limited list of approved foods. Dr. Sebi claimed that for more than 400 years, Western medical science is treating sicknesses incorrectly, with very rare cures being noticed. Sebi claimed that diseases are caused by the host being infected due to treatment practices using chemicals because this technique was adopted inherently flawed in society. As a more effective and intuitive approach, Dr. Sebi disproves this technique by referring to African philosophy, normally called African Bio-mineral Balance. The method promoted by Sebi suggests that if a mucous-membrane gets damaged, diseases are induced in the body. A drastic build-up of this mucus is produced when this happens, which in turn creates a disease. So, what is Sebi's answer or what is the alternate way to cope with the problem?

The prevention of these mucus build-ups issue in the body depends on diet. The famous African Bio-mineral Balance philosophy assumes that illness can occur in an acidic climate only. The remedy recommended by Dr. Sebi is to develop a diet plan that mainly focuses on developing an alkaline deficiency. Like many other modern diets, plants are more concentrated with alkaline; because plants are naturally alkaline.

Dr. Sebi asserts that alkaline diet develops an atmosphere in which infection can not flourish. He also argues that African Bio-mineral-Balance rejuvenates damaged body cell tissue. Dr. Sebi has developed a detoxification cleanse process that will purify every cell of the body. the expectation is that, the human body will begin cell rejuvenation process. His alkaline diet, which is mainly based on the famous theory of African Bio-Mineral was developed by Alfredo Darrington Bowman, also self-educated herbalist known best as Dr. Sebi. Although Sebi was not really a medical doctor and he did not hold any doctorate degree. Without depending on standard Western medicine, Sebi built this diet for everyone who wishes to naturally cure or prevent illness and improve health.

As per Dr. Sebi, sickness in an area of the body is the product of mucus build-up. Build-up of mucus, for instance, is pneumonia, whereas diabetes is excess mucus in the pancreas. He claims that in an alkaline setting, diseases do not exist and start to arise when the body is more acidic. He claims to restore the body's normal alkaline condition and detoxify the infected body by closely observing his routine using his expensive supplements. Originally, Dr. Sebi believed that this diet could treat diseases like HIV, sickle cell anemia, leukemias, and lupus. Sebi's diet contains a detailed list of items that have been approved by Sebi. The diet is considered a "vegan diet" the reason is that animal products are not allowed. Dr.Sebi believed that for a human body to heal itself, one must follow the diet faithfully for the remaining of your life. Finally, while many individuals believe that the program has cured them, no scientific findings support these statements. but still the Sebi diet plans are famous all over the world with many positive reviews available on internet.

1.2 How to start and what are the basic principles of this diet:

Dr. Sebi believed that diseases are the product of increased mucus and more acidity in body; he claimed that diseases will not occur in alkaline climate. His method, which requires a very restricted diet and effective supplements, promises to purify and restore alkalinity levels in the body (no scientific evidence is able to help his promises).

On the website of Sebi, the guidelines of the diet are quite strict and illustrated in details. You must obey these main guidelines, according to Sebi's dietary guide:

Rule 1. Only the foods specified in the dietary guide must be consumed.

Rule 2. Drink 3.8 liters (1 gallon) of water per day.

Rule 3: Take the supplements an hour before medication.

Rule 4: No animal product allowed.

Rule 5: It does not allow any alcohol.

Rule 6: Stop wheat items and consume only the "natural-growing grains" referred to in the guide.

Rule 7: Don't kill your food. Avoid microwave use.

Rule 8: Stop canned fruits or seedless ones.

There seem to be no clear rules on nutrients. Nevertheless, this diet has low protein, as lentils, beans, and animal products are forbidden. For strong muscles, skin, and body joints, protein is an essential nutrient. Besides, Sebi's listed food products, which are nutrients rich and promise to clean your body and replenish your cells, are still expected to be purchased. The "all-inclusive" kit (search on web), which includes 20 different items that are said to purify and heal your body just at the quickest possible rate, is recommended to be purchased. Besides this, no clear guidelines for supplements are given. Instead, you are supposed to order any medication that suits your health concern. Just for example, "Bio Ferro" capsules tend to treat liver problems, cleanses your bloodstream, improve immunity, encourage weight loss, help digestive problems, and enhance overall well-being. Besides, the supplements do not provide a comprehensive list of ingredients or quantities, making it somehow difficult to understand whether they can do what they are supposed to do. The diet limits animal products while, focuses on vegan food, but with far more strict guidelines. It limits seedless fruits. For instance, it only allows Sebi's approved list of "normal growing grains."

Here is a short description of the foods items that his dietary guide recommends:

Vegetables: use amaranth greens, eat sea vegetables, avocado, garbanzo, bell peppers, beans, chayote, cucumber, izote, kale, lettuce (all but iceberg), onions, nopales, okra, olives, zucchini, squash, tomatoes (only cherry and plum), tomatillo, turnip greens, cress, purslane, wild arugula. Vegetables:

Fruits: apples, bananas, berries (all kinds, not cranberries), elderberries, cantaloupe, dates, figs, currants, grapes, lime, mango peaches, oranges, plums, prickly pears, papayas, peaches, pears, prunes, grapes (seeded), light coconut jelly, soursops, tamarind, etc.

Herbal teas: Burdock, elderberry, chamomile, fennel, ginger, raspberry and tila.

Grains: amaranth, fonio, wheat, spelled, tef, wild rice, Kamut, quinoa.

Nuts and seeds: 'tahini' butter of raw sesame seeds, hemp seeds, raw sesame seeds, walnuts, Brazil nuts.

Oils: olive oil (not cooked), coconut oil (not cooked), grape seed oil, sesame oil, hemp oil, avocado oil.

Seasonings /spices: basil, bay leaf, garlic, dill, oregano, savory, estragon, onion powder, thyme, achiote, cayenne, habanero, pure sea salt, sage, seaweed, pure agave syrup, powder, date sugar.

1.3. Advantages and disadvantages of the Doctor Sebi diet

Advantages:

Due to Its heavy focus on a plant-based diet, this is one advantage of the Sebi diet. The diet encourages a huge proportion of fruits and vegetables that are rich in fiber, vitamins, minerals, and plant sources to be eaten.

Significantly lower inflammation & cell proliferation, as well as defenses against many health disorders, have been linked with diets that are rich in fruit content and vegetables. Those who consume seven or even more servings of fruits and veggies each day had a 25% to 31% lower risk of heart-related disease and cancer (based on study of 65,226 individuals).

Moreover, most people do not consume enough dairy food. In a 2017 survey, 9.3 percent and 12.2 percent of individuals met the fruit and veggie guidelines, respectively. Also, the Dr. Sebi diet encourages consuming whole grain food which is rich in fiber and good fats, such as nuts, beans, and vegetable oils. A lower risk of heart disease has been associated with these foods.

Finally, with overall improved diet plan, health can be improved by avoiding and limiting ultra-processed food.

Disadvantages:

This diet is extremely protein deficient: no animal-based products, the eggs, the dairy, even the soy are permitted by Sebi. He limits many other beans and legumes as well. Some hemp seeds, walnuts, natural growing grains, and Brazil nuts are the only things that have some protein in the diet. It can be quite hard to fulfill dietary requirements from these products alone. Protein is a key element of any cell in the human body, and also to help create and heal tissues, the body requires protein. Muscles, skin, blood, and tissue are all an important building block of protein. Nutritional deficiencies and malnourishment can result from constraining major food and nutritional content. While it supports some fruit and veggies, it curiously limits quite a bit of food. It allows for cherry and plum tomatoes, for instance, but no other types. The Iceberg lettuce and the shiitake mushrooms are other types of food that he limits, which makes this diet much more stringent, making it extremely hard to obey.

The primary focus of Sebi is on his products that make big promises that they will "speed up the recovery process" and "rejuvenate and engage intercellular development." Some packages cost well over $1,500 and do not list any nutrient or quantity specifics. This makes it hard to understand what you'll get from his patented blends and also what exactly his supplements contain.

Above all, Dr. Sebi is not a doctor, so there's no evidence-based study to support his statements and directives. his extremely strict dietary recommendations promote the removal of major food groups that can have harmful health effects or, not to forget, can lead to bad relationship to food. It is important to not fall into a dieting conspiracy trap to know the truth and ensure that every diet you adopt is validated by science.

In 1993, after pretending his diet can cure sensitive situations, such as HIV, lupus and leukemia, Dr. Sebi faced litigation. According to Health line, a court asked him to withdraw making such claims. It is crucial to know that there was no PhD obtained by Dr. Sebi. There was also no scientific support for his diet and nutrients. Finally, other unhealthy habits, such as consuming supplements to reach fullness, are promoted by this diet. Since nutrients are not a significant energy source, unhealthy eating habits are guided further by this argument.

Lacks of protein and other key minerals, which are an excellent source of nutrition, are not allowed by Sebi's nutrition guide. Only walnuts, some Brazilian nuts, sesame seeds and hemp seeds that are not rich sources of protein are allowed. For example, 4 grams and 9 grams of protein are given by 1/4 cup (25 grams) of walnuts and 3 tbsp (30 grams) of hemp seeds, accordingly.

You will need to eat incredibly large quantities of such foods to satisfy your protein intake needs. While certain foods, including potassium, beta carotene, and vitamin-C and Vitamin-E, appear high in foods in diet, they are relatively low in omega3, iron, calcium, and vitamin D and B12, the common nutrients of concern to those who adopt a strictly limited plant-based diet. Dr. Sebi's website mentions that in his products, some ingredients are patented and not specified. This is important, as it is unclear which nutrition you get and how much you get, it make difficult to know if you will fulfill your daily nutrient requirements. Another significant issue with Dr. Sebi's diet policy is the lack of objective evidence to support it, not based on actual research.

He mentions that acid development in your body is regulated by the foods and supplements mentioned in his food. In order to hold PH level of blood between 7.36 and 7.44, the body strictly controls the acid-base balance, naturally rendering the body mildly alkaline. Blood pH will go out of that range in extreme cases, such as ketoacidosis from diabetic conditions. Without instant medical treatment, this can be devastating.

The Sebi plan has no actual evidence to support its arguments, like so many other diet fads (GM diet, here's watching you), Taub-Dix says. Not only diet mainly depend on supplements marketed by the firm, but even names are misleading, as there are currently no credentials or qualifications for Dr. Sebi (whose real name is "Alfredo Bowman") exist.

"Taub-Dix says," I agree that Sebi's name almost gives the diet legitimacy or enables you think it's a reliable diet because he's just not a physician at all. "Another point is that, in case you have advice on what to buy, you need to be aware of every diet where someone sells something to you, such as supplements." Moreover, according to Taub-Dix, the diet's promises of detoxifying and curing the system are deceptive and potentially dangerous. Your liver functions and kidneys are already in very good at eliminating toxins from the body, but there is no evidence that, according to the Mayo Clinic, any foods or drugs can either assist or impede this process.

The key fear of Taub-Dix is that "healing" promises of the plan will lead certain individuals who are treating a disease to follow the diet as a substitute for their drugs that can be harmful. If you're trying to manage a condition, before making significant decisions about your medications or diet, be sure to consult with a doctor.

The doctor Sebi's plan will probably leave you struggling short in terms of your nutrition, especially when proteins are involved. Although the diet allows for nuts and seeds that might have some nutrient content, the total lack of animal foods would likely leave you nutrition-deficient as per Taub-Dix.

Although it may be possible to manage your protein intake on a diet focused on plants, it can be difficult to do so. And the restriction of animal products (such as tofu or vegetarian burgers, for instance) and nutrients outside the diet's own product by the Dr. Sebi diet will make it much harder.

According to H. Chan the School Public Health, on average, a person needs almost 7 g of protein per Twenty pounds of body weight every day. So, you can eat about 56 g of protein daily if you reach 160 pounds. For background, as per the USDA's Food-Data Central, a 1-ounce portion of Sebi-approved walnuts provides just over Four grams of protein. You can also be left lacking in omega-3 fatty acids by limiting animal products, Taub-Dix says. Omega-3s, according to the Penn State Milton S. Hershey Medical Center, are critical for brain function, which contributes to your memory. Deficiency cans results to symptoms such as tiredness, poor memory and dry skin.

Dr. Sebi's diet plan also prevents all processed foods, as per

Taub-Dix, which is also not necessarily a positive thing. Generally, super-processed foods do not have significant health benefits, but the processed foods could be part of the safe and balanced diet, such as canned fruit or vegetables. They aren't just convenient, readily accessible and easy to prepare with, making meal preparation even more feasible, but most of these packaged foods are also filled with nutrients that the average person might not have been likely to get from their normal dietary habits, Taub-Dix says.

While the focus of Dr. Sebi's diet on adding plenty of fruit and veggies is undoubtedly a positive feature of an otherwise deficient regimen, Taub-Dix says this is not a diet that will have many advantages. It is not a bad thing to add more whole foods, but it is difficult to get the range of ingredients your body requires because of the excessively stringent nature of this approach.

It is important to prioritize the advice of a health care provider, especially for all those aiming at Dr. Sebi's plan to reduce or alleviate a disease or illness. It is best to consult with a doctor before attempting some kind of diet to make sure it is a good plan for you.

Finally, research has also shown that your food may alter your urine pH slightly and temporarily, but not the pH of the blood. Thus, adopting the diet of Dr. Sebi would not make any difference in the long term.

Chapter 2: Foods recommended by Dr. Sebi.

2.1 List of foods approved by Dr. Sebi (food groups)

The Sebi's Diet is purely based on a vegan diet the program focuses on the whole diet based on plants. It emphasizes foods which have been classified as alkaline by Dr. Sebi. It implies that certain plant-based foods (shown below) are not permitted to be consumed. It is important to be on the authorized food list for all the foods you can eat when following this diet plan. Food list by Dr. Sebi with approved food items is given below.

Vegetables: Asparagus, Cucumbers, Squash, Chickpeas, Amaranth greens, Mushrooms (except Shitake), Onions, Olives, Bell peppers, Amaranth Okra, Avocado, Purslane, atones (cherry and plum only), Dandelion greens Sea vegetables, (Wakame/Dulce/Arame/Hijiki/Nori), Chayote, Tom Tomatillo, Garbanzo beans, Turnip greens Kale, Watercress, Lettuce (except for Iceberg), Wild arugula, Mexican squash, Zucchini.

Fruits: Apples, Pears, Figs, Seeded, Cherries, Prunes, Mango, Soft Jelly Coconuts, Cantaloupe, Seeded key limes, Cactus fruit, (Latin or West Indian markets), Papayas, Tamarind, Plums, Seeded grapes, raisins, Bananas, Peaches, Currants, Seeded melons, Oranges, Soursops.

Nuts: Raw Sesame "Tahini" Butter, Brazil nuts, Hemp seed, raw sesame seeds, Walnuts.

Herb: Achiote, Basil, Onion powder Oregano, Bay leaf, Sage, Habanero Cloves, Sweet basil, Dill, Savory, Cayenne Thyme, Tarragon.

Oils: Hemp seed oil, Avocado oil, Coconut oil (not cooked), Grapeseed oil, Olive oil (not cooked), Sesame oil.

Grains: Amaranth, Rye, Chamomile, Burdock, Ginger, Red raspberry, Quinoa, Wild rice, Herbal teas, Fonio, Spelt, Kamut, Tef Anise, Fennel, Elderberry, Tila, Salt, you may consume the pure sea salt with diet or powdered granulated seaweed.

Sweeteners: Alkaline sweeteners. On this food intake, sugar is not permitted, but some alkaline sugar substitutes are allowed. Date glucose (from dried dates) and natural cactus agave syrup can be eaten.

Non – GMO Foods:

You should concentrate on foods derived from plants that are untreated or minimally processed. Also, the foods ones eat must be non-GMO. Used to prevent pesticides and other additives applied to non-organic foods, it is safer to consume organic-food as much of it as possible. As soon as the foods of preference meet the above requirements, they are likely to eventually allow in diet of Dr. Sebi.

The Doctor Sebi food list was considered by some dieters to be much restrictive for their taste. Nevertheless, faithful adherents of the diet believe that inside the list there are still enough foods to enable you to have a variety. A traditional Dr. Sebi diet menu might look like veggies pan-seared on either a bed of wild rice, in avocado oil, or a broad green salad with a seasoning of olive oil as well as a hint of agave syrup. Although that can take some time to become used to it, the food checklist of Dr. Sebi could be easy to stick to and follow for a healthy diet plan.

2.2. Foods you should never eat (and why)

Below are the main foods items that need to be avoiding when following Dr. Sebi's diet:

All types of meat, fish and seafood, Eggs, Wheat, Dairy products, Fast foods, Sugar, Seedless fruits, Garlic, Corn (and product containing corn), All types food that has been processed, GMO foods, any foods that contains artificial food colors and flavors, foods with preservatives and any type of added vitamins or minerals, Soy, Poultry, all food items that contains yeast and baking powder, Alcohol is strictly prohibited.

As this is a nutritional plan that excludes certain groups of foods, it is essential to use particular nutrients in your diet. Broadly speaking, you might need vitamins including B-12 vitamins, as well as some other vitamins and minerals, like iron, omega-3 fatty acid and calcium, etc. However, you can get plenty of them from plant-based diet if you choose them wisely and consume more than one form of plant origin in a single meal. Or you may order Dr. Sebi items, which had some herbs and minerals that will offer you vitamins that are lacking in your diet, but visit your physician before trying them. The orders can be placed via Amazon.

2.3. List of herbs Doctor Sebi: Green Food plus, Sea Moss, Viento and others.

I love how herbal tea consumption has resulted in my general well-being. They help me retain a well-balanced body and have supported one's body to recover itself. Each body is distinct and

different herbs will solve the same problem that you might have in various ways, so I recommend that you should do your own research-work and communicating with an herbalist (who understands the African Bio-Mineral Balance) even if you're an herbal medicine specialist or have a name for a disease. Following are also the plants I like to use for repair, in no precise order.

1. Sea Moss-in conjunction with Bladderwrack, I normally

drink it. use hemp milk some dates, and cloves to make a special drink from it. 92 out of 102 minerals composing the human body are found in it. I like it wet. It serves to remind myself to Milo, kind of thing. I prefer to drink it in the morning and in the evening. Also, I utilize it several times per week to cleanse my face. I simply use spring water to incorporate a dime-sized quantity of powder, end up making it like a paste and spread this over my face. Around 5 mins or more, I keep it on, and rinse. * Try regularly our multi-mineral, Cell which helps you, if you don't really like the taste of Sea Moss.

Dr. Sebi also often spoke favorably for sea moss; it's almost a common diet item that is a part of daily life for all of us who adopt his diet. He said that, there is still seems to be uncertainty about it which sort of seaweed (species) are called "Irish moss" and how much nutritional value they have. a "Today, however, Ireland sea moss, nod simple moss may be referred to as a variety of various seaweeds, like (but probably not restricted to) Kappaphycus, Chondrus crispus, alvarezii (a.k.a Eucheuma cottonii) as well as various species inside the genus Gracilaria, based on where you live on the planet.

Gigartinales, Chondrus crispus and cymbopogon alvarezii refer to the same group, but Gracilaria refers to the group of Gracilariales.

K. Alvarezii belongs to a group called Solieriaceae. In contrast, the Chondrus crispus belongs to Gigartinaceae's family, and Gracilaria refers to the group of Gracilariaceae. Seaweed naming convention utilizes the naming system, a "two-term naming scheme."

Knowing this helps to classify the genus to which a certain species belongs, from their name alone. The group to which the species belongs is identified by the first part of its name, whereas the second section describes the species inside the group, i.e. species belongs to the genus Chondrus is Chondrus crispus. In colder waters, Chondrus crispus develops and occurs in excess around the mountainous parts of the Europe's Atlantic coasts, particularly Ireland and the United Kingdom, and Iceland. It can be located on the Canadian and North American Atlantic coasts.

It has a smooth and cartilages consistency in its moist and natural state and it may have different colors from greenish-yellow to red or dark purple to purple-brown. It does have a pale yellow or

translucent color when cleaned and sun-dried, which is typically how this will look once you buy the dried plant.

2. Dandelion Root: While I have never been a real hardcore coffee addict, I prepare Dandelion Root Tea that tastes quite like coffee whenever I want to feel the flavor. Introduce Hemp-Milk with Date Syrup and then you've created a latte for yourself. What's really incredible about it, this is also a liver cleanser. Cleaning up the liver offers you some vitality in

return. So, consuming this in morning is indeed a perfect substitute for coffee and helps the body to stay in detox mode rather than having all the acid with in the body which coffee drinking can generate.

3. Damiana: I drink Damiana whenever I feel mentally unbalanced, anxious or nervous. Even though it is marketed as an herbal remedy, it helps me feel relaxed and not excited. Still, the experience might be unique for others. A perfect tea when you're having menstruation. Try Nerves Support in-case you are searching for a treatment that can assist you with anxiety and depression.

4-5 Burdock Root and Combo Sarsaparilla-Burdock Root contains up to 102 minerals at low concentrations in the body. To offer me a mineral boost, I want to mix this with other herbs. Because Sarsaparilla contains the highest amount of iron and works as a magnet for minerals, I always combine them (usually, like Linden Flower, with a third herb that rounds out the flavor).

6. Yellow Dock: I introduce this to the tea combos when my skin may feel out of whack, indicating my lymphatic system feels overwhelmed or I have a rash with something I have affected (or touched me). It doesn't always taste fine on its own. I even grind it up and prepare a face mask out of it in a coffee grinder (adding it mainly to Sea Moss).

7. Blue Vervain: When I feel lacking in magnesium, I drink

this. Indications of this are that my brain is overdriving to one problem, and I cannot "wind it off" or I cannot sleep. That relieves anxiety. I typically take-out supplement for Nerve-Support in capsule form, since it tastes like a metallic chemical that's not perfect. But I can mix it with Damiana or Linden as a tea that has a light floral taste. * Aside-MANY people who routinely smoke marijuana are seriously deficient in magnesium.

8. Cascara Sagrada: - This is what I call 'Boo Boo Tea,' lmao. I go straight for this, if I'm constipated. It also doesn't taste amazing, but I equate this to brown alcohol. I often get a couple of shots. I recommend drinking it at night, so I'll be ready to go in the morning. I do not recommend drinking it and then moving out for a long period where you'll have to use a toilet in someone else's home. If so, I would suggest covering the smell from some of the Bathroom Drops,

particularly if you consumed some junk in the first place to become constipated.

9. Elderberry: When I have been around sick people, and I'd like to give some boost to immunity, Elderberry pushes my immune system in hyperdrive. But be careful. You can get extremely nauseous when you eat too much Elderberry. Also-to get them more appealing, a perfect complement to other herbs.

10. Linden Flower: These are perfect for lung mucus expulsion. Truly calming. When we feel dry throat or a constant cough, it's my time to go. It has a floral taste that is mild. Great compliment to herbal extracts with strong flavors to round out.

11. BLACK WALNUT: Normally used to treat parasitic worms, like diphtheria and syphilis, and certain other diseases. It is used for leukemia as well. Some individuals use Black Walnut mostly as gargle, apply this as a hair dye into the scalp, or place this on skin in order to treat wounds.

12. Chickweed: use this thing for constipation, stomach & bowel issues and blood disorders along with asthma and other lung-related diseases. It can be used for scurvy and psoriasis as well as scratching, and muscle & joint pain as an enzyme inhibitor. For skin conditions, including boils, sores and ulcers, it can be applied to the skin.

13. NETTLE: is used for hair growth stimulation. In individuals with diabetes, it helps regulate blood sugar. It decreases gingivitis-related bleeding, treats kidney and helps in recovering urinary tract disorders, and offers water retention. It prevents and handles diarrhea.

14. Mugwort: To induce digestive juices and bile secretion, mugwort is used. It is frequently used to prevent digestive tract diseases and to help with all digestive system issues and

is said to have an anti-fungal effect. It has antibacterial, expectorative and antiasthmatic properties. It can be used in the treatment of a wide range of infectious diseases, like tapeworm, roundworm, and thread-worm. Mugwort is thought to be successful. For irregular cycles and other menstrual issues, females take mugwort. It is sometimes used as a tonic for the liver; for circulation promotion; and as a sedative. If pregnant, do not use) *.

15. Sage: For digestive issues, including lack of appetite, gas, stomach pain, diarrhea, bloating, and heartburn, SAGE can be used. It can also be used for minimizing transpiration & saliva increased production; for depression, memory loss & Alzheimer's disease. It has been used by women for painful menstrual cycles, to fix irregular milk flow during breastfeeding, and to minimize menopausal hot flashes.

16. Sarsaparilla: For the prevention of gout, gonorrhea, open sores, rheumatoid arthritis, pain in joints, cough, fever, high blood pressure, skin diseases, and indigestion, sarsaparilla is considered effective. It also has the maximum (according to Dr. Sebi) iron content of any herb.

17. Strawberry leaf: The main use of Strawberries Leaves is to alleviate gastrointestinal discomfort and joint pain. They include essential minerals, such as iron, an important component of production of red blood cells, and hemoglobin, which helps to support anemia. It helps in reducing high

blood pressure due to its vasodilating effects. It is also advertised as a blood purifier and provides relief from mucus.

18. Bladderwrack: is a type of kelp which is used as a therapeutic strategy for obesity and cellulite to activate the thyroid gland. It is rich in iodine and helps to improve the metabolism. It also decreases inflammation, improves muscles, enhances circulation, it protects the skin, supports vision, and prevents premature ageing; also it reduces cancer risk, and improves heart health.

In your search for a healthy body, I hope the list provided above will helps you. It's a recommendation I want to make to take each herb one at a time and to learn how each one makes you feel personally. Reading books and listening to people is fine, but finding it out by yourself helps you with a more intimate view about what is good for you.

2.4. The shopping list of Doctor Sebi's approved products

So, you've got Dr. Sebi's Dietary Guidance on board, and you're happy to shop? Few things are fairly easy to locate, but you will have to look a little harder for few others. You will have to search beyond the model you're used to for conventional food stores or the big box stores whether you're searching for organic or herbal goods or grains.

Taking the bananas that are approved, such as orange, burro, and baby bananas. You might buy one of these in a normal grocery shop, and you'll notice a bunch more of what you need for this Serbian diet plan if you search a little deeper.

Vegetables: According to Dr. Sebi "Never use the microwave, this will kill all your food."

Amaranth greens, Bell Peppers, a variety of Spinach, Dandelion greens, Cucumber, Avocado, Burro Banana, Asparagus, Chayote (Mexican Squash), Jicama, Garbanzo beans (chickpeas), Izote "cactus flower/ cactus leaf," Kale, Lettuce (all, but not Iceberg), Mushrooms (all, but not Shitake), Mustard greens, Olives, Onions, Okra, Squash, Nopales (Mexican Cactus), Poke salad –greens, Spinach (use sparingly), String beans, Tomato –only cherry and plum, Tomatillo, Turnip greens,

Zucchini, Sea Vegetables (dulse / wakame /arame/ nori/ hijiki).

Fruits: "No canned and seedless fruits". Dr. Sebi.

Apples, Bananas (only the smallest one are allowed or the Burro (mid-size original banana), Berries complete variety Elderberries in any form (but no cranberries), Cherries, Currants, Figs, Dates, Grapes –seeded, Cantaloupe, Mango, Limes, Orange, Melons, Peaches, Pears, Plums, Prunes, Papayas, Raisins –seeded, Soft Jelly Coconuts, Soursops, Sugar apples- chermoya.

Herbal Teas: Alvaca, Chamomile, Anise, Cloves, Ginger, Lemongrass, Red Raspberry, Sea Moss Tea, Fennel

Spices & Seasonings: Mild Flavors, Bay leaf, Cilantro, Basil, Marjoram, Oregano, Tarragon, Sweet Basil, Thyme, Achiote, Cayenne, Cumin, Coriander, Onion Powder, Sage, Dill, Salty Flavors, Pure Sea Salt, Powdered Granulated Seaweed, Kelp/Dulce.

Sweet Flavors: Pure Maple Syrup only B grade is recommended, Maple "Sugar" (derived from maple syrup), Date "Sugar" (derived from dates), Pure Agave Syrup derived from cactus.

Nuts & Seeds: Raw Almonds, Almond Butter, Raw Sesame, Raw Sesame Seeds, "Tahini" Butter, and Walnuts/Hazelnut.

It is surprising that people have "allergies with wheat", reason behind it's not a natural grain; it is produced by science and is a hybrid product, and it is acid-based.

Natural Growing Grains have a nature of alkaline-based foods; it is therefore recommended that you must use the following products instead of Wheat:

Black Rice, Amaranth, Quinoa, Rye, Spelt, Tef, Wild Rice, Kamut.

Chapter 3: Dr. Sebi's diet for management of various diseases

3.1. Dr. Sebi's diet with diabetes and herpes

Dr. Sebi's remedy to cure Diabetes is straightforward and needs to have very little money, but few will obey his plan. His idea was quite easy. Only stop eating.

Many people tend to get their foot chopped off before they even have to stop eating. Yet in 27 days during fasting, Dr. Sebi healed his own diabetes. Remember we discuss in the introduction that Sebi was a self-educated man and he was diagnosed with diabetes.

Many people have also published the same findings. One person on You-Tube also confirmed that he successfully treated his diabetes by following Dr. Sebi's fasting program.

Dr. Sebi stated, "Mucus is really the source of all types of disease, and mucus falls only after you've absorbed anything that shouldn't have in your bloodstream."

Dr. Sebi's strategy is to rid the body of needless mucosa, which is considered the origin of all diseases. He states this: "Our study indicates that any type of disorder has its origin when mucous membrane becomes weakened. i.e. whether there is excess mucous inside the bronchial tubes, the resulting disease will relates to bronchitis; if it is found in inside the lungs, the resultant disease will be known as pneumonia; and inside pancreatic duct, the resultant issue will simply be diabetes; mucous in the joints called arthritis.

Besides, the mucosa in the retina causes blindness; if observed across the thyroid gland, the same will result in thyroid cancer. Basically, the illness will occur in the body whenever this stagnant poison is build up in the body.

The healing diet can be found mentioned below it's important to remember that Sebi has suggested foods mentioned here for recovery from a disease for more than 30 years. Suppose your favorite food is absent from our list. In that case, we assure you that based on our research and findings, it has little nutritious benefit and could be harmful to your health; that is the reason we have neglected that and not included in our list of approved food items.

So, what if you have MUCUS build up in your body?

If you do have diabetes, you might've got mucus in the pancreatic duct. Thus, part of the procedure (fasting) is to eliminate the mucus. His mother took 57 days of fasting to clear the mucus. For this moment, Dr. Sebi must have kept her peaceful and quiet. I fasted on four different occasions,

most of which were 12 days, and then on my last fast, I saw no mucus at all.

The really nice herbal tea for mucus that I created is Elder-berry tea, The Red Raspberry and Black Walnut Leaves or Burdock. Take a full tablespoon of every herb and put them all in one & half liters of fresh spring water and wait to boil the water. Boil the herbal tea for about 15 minutes, and then include another half-liter of water. Get the herbal tea to an-other boil again and then remove from stove. Strain all the herbs and set all of them aside for use for upcoming days. On next day, you can reuse the extracted herbs again. You may put the herbal tea in carafe or you may store it inside the re-frigerator so that it may be consumed later on. Drink the tea for whole day as required.

Besides fasting, you need to continue with Dr. Sebi Verified Diet Schedule and monitor your diet closely. There are many other things you must care for that will help with diabetes, too.

Mulberry-Leaves and Black-Seeds are the most recom-mended replacements. Black Seeds have been studied and proven that only little amount of them let say only 2 tea-spoons in single day is enough to cure diabetes.

Figleaves are known as the best-selling leaf today in the mar-ket commonly used for curing diabetes according to a survey published in 1998. Mulberry leaves are also the number one treatment used by diabetic patients in the Middle East. You can simply add some black seeds to your herbal teas too.

Some useful items are Swiss chard, Sour melon, Garlic, avocado, Okra, Ginseng, Fenugreek and Red Clover.

3.2. Herpes

Having a series of fasting or consuming food items that are much less toxic to the electrical body would undoubtedly aim to rid everyone of herpes. The purpose is to build an atmosphere in which the cause of the disease cannot survive. Your cells are in search of oxygen. Toxins such as medicines for herpes will steal the oxygen from cells, which, in most instances, will tie with herpes.

Healing herpes is going to be taking some cleaning and plant-based Iron products. Implement the same way we are doing to cure HIV. You're going to start with Iron Plus with Bio Ferro.

Plus Powder (Bromide for tea)

The key to success is NUTRITION. Although the immune response is getting Support from iron, much of the mineral nutrients required will come from bromide plus powder; you just have to make the tea then drink it. Boil some water, pour into a small blender, turn it on, introduce about one teaspoon of bromide, and let it mix for a couple of minutes. Do so twice or more than once a day.

A perhaps a more significant way of treating herpes is dealing with foods that you shouldn't bring in your mouth and the body. Stay out of the starches and sweets. Very minimal portions of fruit or vegetable food are sweet. Have more bitter food than sweet food. However, there is a lot of lettuce to choose from, however. For healing reasons but stay away from avocados and chickpeas, avoid quinoa and gravitate and move towards more zucchini, use squash, cactus flower or leaf.

If you already have plant-based iron green tea such as the burdock, the dandelion, the yellow dock, that will surely help. Consume as many days as you are able to; a minimum of ten days. You don't have to mix it. That's your choice if you want to. Depending upon where you are, they can be challenging to locate. You might need to order these roots through online herbal websites. (Already mentioned in the previous section).

Practice fasting; prepare to get on with it. The more fasting you have, the more chances of healing you will have.

If you're feeling weak, eat some dates. They're sweet, but they're not supposed to agitate your cells. Eat just when you are weak.

You may have salads just like you were enjoying a bag full of potato chips. Get a crisp light (but no iceberg lettuce). The response to what Sebi tries to teach us is to get rid of mucus build up in the body, and it ends up going like this:

There is just one disorder, and this is the product of the mucous membrane being damaged. The mucous membrane is important to preserve health as it is that membrane which covers the cells. If you tear down the mucous layer, it transforms into pus and reveals the cells.

i.e., Sickle Cell Anemia happens when blood plasma is broken and turns to sickle by a mucous membrane. The mucus falls in the plasma and into the cell itself, splits and dis-unifies the cell. By removing the mucous, the cell get unites again. You need to feed a patient with massive amounts of iron phosphate to sustain that amount. Not iron oxide.

Iron-based herbal substances developed by Dr. Sebi, like Iron Plus or Bio Ferro, supply the body from over 14 primary organic (carbon-hydrogen-oxygen) plants and herbal minerals.

A collection of vegetation cell-based food items includes Iron Phosphate, but are extracted from electrically activated tropical plants; some originate from tropical Africa and Honduras. Also, some belong to the Caribbean; others might be from Latin American countries.

Herbal plants in Dr. Sebi's vegetation-based cell food are strongly electrical. Their molecular structures are complete, and it's based on carbon. They would quickly assimilate and energies the human body with foods served by nature to us. The nutrients provide your body with the requisite phosphates and carbonates along with iodides and bromide ... also called the food of life!

3.3. Liver cleansing with the diet of Dr. Sebi

You may have read of allopathic medications' adverse effects because most of them are moderate acne, digestive problems or nausea, right? Several researchers have eventually demonstrated that consuming so many allopathic medications clearly influences the kidneys and liver. Now, you're also supposed to think beyond acne and nausea problems, and this isn't all the allopathic drugs that can do with you. If you depend on unnecessary drugs, you are at risk. Various variables lead to this durability. But even though you realize that your liver is in trouble because of the fast cure medications that you take, you're always doing the same thing; you're certainly at fault. This implies that you don't even trust your long-term wellbeing. We're going to look at Sebi's liver disease treatment kit and its advantages, but before going for that, let me remind you one thing most of you are reading this book because of allopathic medications. These medications, which we also term modern medicine, have rendered Dr. Sebi's cure kit for the liver necessary for about all. In simple words, you'll see why and how to see some of the components in Sebi's liver disease cure package.

Sebi's Liver Diseases Treatment Kit includes:

Punarnavadi Mandoor: It is a combination of Punarnava and many other herbs, which have hepatoprotective nature. The first component in Dr. Sebi's liver disorder cure package is a blend of up to one dozen herbs. Both these herbs are obtained from their native lands.

Sutsekhar Ras Gold: It is a Fine powder of Shuddha Parada (known as Herbal distilled Mercury). Swarna Bhasma, (known as Bhasma of Gold), Tankana Bhasma (called Borax), The Tamra Bhasma (It is prepared from Copper), The Gandhaka (you may call it Purified and processed Sulphur), Shuddha Vatsanabha (maybe known as Purified Aconitum Ferox), and Shankha Bhasma (It is a Conch Shell which is processed, purified and combined to make Sutshekhar ras gold. These things are known as the ashes of metals that are purified to make Sure that these strong metals may only contain the healing properties in them.

Chandrakala Ras: It is another herbal formula that is a natural combination of uncommon herbs and solid minerals. Ela (Cardamom), Amla, Camphor, Jatiphala, and Shalmali are among the well-known herbal ingredients for Chandrakanta-ras. So, this herbal combination is required if you want to maintain the liver intact.

Punarnava Herbal blend: Since the punarnava is among the best herbs that we have for curing liver problems, Sebi wants to use it against all liver diseases. Also, to improve the overall health of the liver in particular. These ingredients used in it are a blend of many herbs. These herbs used here will differ based on different liver disorders you may be suffering from.

Sarphunka Plant: This is known as a plant's scientific name, and Dr. Sebi used it to cope with multiple liver disorders. Not just that, it holds a unique spot in Ayurveda's ancient healing science. Because of its unmatched role in curing liver disease, that is included in Dr. Sebi's liver disease cure kit.

AHP Zinc Powder: Liver probably is the most essential organ in the human body. Liver contains too many enzymes and hormones along with components that are essential for our body to perform many functions. It detoxifies different metabolites and generates enzymes, produces synthesizes proteins, and makes the biochemicals required for digestion. These are only few of the liver's activities, and, besides, they have an indirect effect on human well-being when they involve the operation of the digestive tract and the gall bladder. Since the liver has too many irreplaceable functions, and too many other body organs are directly based on it, you mustn't neglect it anymore. The first most thing you can do if you frequently consume antibiotics and allopathic medicines for any reason, make sure to get your liver screened. If you've already completed the test and, sadly, there are any complications, you can just order Dr. Sebi's liver disorder cure package. You can buy all the kits online by searching on Google or follow "drsebihealing.com."

Benefits of Dr. Sebi Package for Curing Liver disease.

There are so many liver diseases cured using Dr. Sebi's liver disease cure package. For example, the following liver diseases are causing problems for millions of human beings. Luckily, we can easily get rid of them by using just the herbal solution provided by Dr. Sebi. The following are the main issues cured by using Dr. Sebi's Kit for Liver diseases.

- Cancer of the liver

- Liver with fat on it

- Hepatitis A, Hepatitis B, and Hepatitis C

- Cirrhosis of liver

- Diseases across the Gall's bladder

- Pancreas-related disorders

These issues and several other health problems may be resolved by using Dr. Sebi's liver disorder cure kit, and they are closely linked to the Liver. Besides, the toxicity introduced by improper usage

of allopathic medications may also be reduced. And it just costs $160 to allow the use of all these opportunities. Yes, in just $160, you can get a complete and comprehensive solution against all the major liver problems. Besides the herbs and other herbal mixtures, which are recommended by Dr. Sebi, you may get a plan to alter your diet plan and lifestyle. Dr. Sebi has always believed in keeping the food safe for the body.

So, with Sebi's kit for curing your liver, you'll even get clear guidance about how you may use it and any other improvements you need to make in your lifestyle to hold your liver condition in control. You can place an order for your pack from "drsebihealing.com" now. Please notice that Dr. Sebi's liver cure kit would last for only two months, so this is probably the lowest time required by your liver to use these herbal medicines kit. Also, unlike the other Sebi's kits, you may customize the kit according to your liver problem. Upon your check-out process, you will then be required to provide some basic information regarding your disease along with the issues you face. Herbal doctors will tailor the Sebi's liver disease care package specifically for your body and its issues.

3.4. The best electric foods and herbs Dr. Sebi for hypertension

When walls of the vessels are crossed, or plaqued and get stuffed, the blood flow is reduced when it flows from the heart towards the aorta; hence pressure is produced by the arteries; hence blood pressure rises and becomes greater than normal above the point typically meant to be, the resulting consequence is, hypertension (also known high blood pressure) has formed.

Diet is at the top when it comes to the causes of high blood pressure, particularly in the United States. It has been reported in a study that over 85% of cases of high blood pressure are directly linked to bad dieting habits. In every age group and gender, African Americans are reported to

have more cases of high blood pressure than other US races. High blood pressure may result in other diseases like strokes, large heart than normal, artery coronary diseases, typhoid fever, tonsillitis, scarlet fever, and often kidney diseases. These diseases are likely to have high blood pressure (known as hypertension, too) among Afro-Americans.

3.5. What is considered as a high blood pressure situation?

Suppose you want to measure the blood pressure. In that case, all you need is a tool called blood pressure gauge or B.P apparatus, which is also called a sphygmomanometer which is capable of recording two types of information regarding Blood Pressure: the 1st one is known as the systolic, it is the higher reading whereas 2nd one is known as the diastolic, and is considered as lower reading.

Therefore, diastolic may be considered less problematic than systolic elevated blood pressure readings since systolic unveils the pressure built up by blood when it is pumped from the heart towards the aorta right before it passes into the passageways inside the arteries. When the systolic reading becomes high, blood pressure is deemed high. Also, the arteries' walls become clogged and there become plaques inside the walls that impede blood flow. Under normal situations, the reading of systolic high blood pressure ranges from 120-150 millimeters. On the other hand, a high reading, let say 140/190, points towards high blood pressure and any reading over 180/115, maybe even more.

What are the causes of high blood pressure?

High blood pressure situations are induced by consuming food that creates plaque that clogs around the arteries' wall while the blood circulating inside the arteries is high, thereby causing increased pressure inside the arteries throughout the circulation process. From the heart to other body organs, the blood flows directly from the heart towards the aorta and arteries. The blood supply in the arteries' corridors is suppressed when walls of the arteries become narrow, and they get hardened due to heavy plaque-induced by poor dieting.

Another thing to keep up in mind is that when a person's age is increased, the arteries automatically get hardened because many times the diet is poor. When people get older, this triples the risk of triggering and causing high blood pressure.

High blood pressure is caused by:

Apart from the hardening and clogging of arteries owing to the inadequate blood supply, which

may cause elevated blood pressure. Synthetic medications,

fatty foods, and harmful patterns of behavior trigger elevated blood pressure: the following are also cases of high blood pressure.

Stress, Tobacco, Aging, Bad diet is also a very important cause: many coffees, Fried and oily foods items and other processed foods and Overeating.

High blood pressure Symptoms:

Dr. Sebi' sees the effects of high blood pressure as the "navy seal sniper attacker," and there are hardly any visible indicators of high blood pressure. This does not indicate, though, that there are no complications. The only visible signs of high blood pressure are difficulty in breathing; the eyes can get distorted; a headache can arise?

A person claimed that one of his aunts had elevated blood pressure. Her blood pressure signs were dizziness and that her heartbeat was fasting. "But, because signs of high blood pressure are not often apparent, it received a reputation as the" sniper killer of the navy seal.

Dr. Sebi's recommended diet for curing High blood pressure:

"All the elevated blood pressure medications imitate water; hence it's a common-sense that you ought to consume plenty of freshwaters," hence you need to consume pure spring water.

Low blood pressure medicine causes thinning of the blood, so that drinking water thins the blood. Divide the weight by 2, so consume the sum of ounces of water. For starters, you'd break 150/2, which is 75 ounces of water a day, if you weigh 150.

Eating five separate kinds of fruits and vegetables in a day will help avoid clogging of the arteries and help to avoid shut down of artery walls and of plaque deposits. Asparagus, broccoli, onions, seeded grapes, oranges, and peaches are some common fruits and vegetables rich in antioxidants that help resist artery walls and plaques; you may see the diet guide for more help on natural fruits and veggies to cure high blood pressure.

Potassium-rich diets are helpful since potassium encourages the body to release sodium to cope with high blood pressure issues. Eat mostly potassium-rich fruits and vegetables like small red-potatoes, whereas stop salty foods. See the dietary guide for more details, as mentioned above.

Fruits and vegetables rich in fiber are good for curing high blood pressure; as they can relieve pressure, which helps to eliminate waste that has been sucked around the artery walls.

High blood pressure may be experienced after eating:

Most of the cases of High blood pressure are recorded after eating. It is critical because after you have eaten something, it is difficult to know its causes. You need to recognize what things to eliminate that could be dangerous to increasing your blood pressure. These are lethal to your good health but what you should not consume is as important as what you should consume. When eating, you do not want to get elevated blood pressure. Stop the following foods:

Particularly if the meal is called a nutritious meal, stop overheating.

Don't consume a salty meal, but keep clear of the salt. Inside the walls of arteries, salt transforms and activates plaque. In general, these foods include salt, but please read the label placed on foods you consume to prevent sodium intake: avoid soda, baking soda, soy sauce, meat tenderizers, and monosodium glutamate (MSG).

Lots of meat, candy, baked products, and cakes. Stop them all. Don't buy any frozen goods, which stands with fruits and vegetables, making sure you don't buy canned food. Eat nothing produced with milk, really rich in salt, and no cheese at all, yogurt, and alcohol are prohibited. Take out dairy items from your diet. Do not eat very late in the evening,

Do not consume rice. Instead, eat brown and wild rice in case you do so.

3.6. Dr. Sebi's recommended food for curing Hypertension

Dr. Sebi proposes the following herbs as they open up the blood vessels and arteries' wall and remove plaques from the artery wall. These herbs rich in minerals are organic electric herbs of alkaline origin. They have been investigated and have proved to be great sources of treatment for hypertension. Herbal herbs are typically strong in strength, so much of them for the blood would be heavy in strength. Here is the list:

- Black cohosh

- Basil

- Yellow dock

- Cayenne

- Oregano

- Fennel

3.7. How to lose weight by following your diet

Condition like Overweight and having obesity are characterized as the accumulation of abnormal or unnecessary fat that poses a health danger. The body to mass index or (BMI), is called the weight of an individual (in kgs) divided by square of height (in meters), is a crude population obesity metric. Generally, a person having a BMI of 30 or above is deemed obese. It is deemed overweight by an individual with a BMI equal to or greater than 25.

Overweight and obesity significantly contribute to diabetes, coronary disorders and cancer, and a variety of chronic diseases. But being overweight and having obesity were once considered a concern only for countries with high-income. Still, now it's rising significantly in low or middle-income countries, especially urban ones.

Dr. Sebi's diet discourages the Western lifestyle, which is rich in highly processed foods filled with salt, fat, sugar, and calories. Dr. Sebi encourages an unprocessed diet plan instead of processed foods. Many that adopt a plant-based diet appear to have a lower incidence of obesity and cardiac disease than the Western diet.

A 12-month survey of 65 individuals showed that those who adopted an unrestricted, low fat, plant-based, whole-food diet lost dramatically more weight than those who did not adopt the diet. Those on Sebi's diet lost, on average about 26.6 pound (12.1 kgs) at the six-month point, compared to 3.5 pounds or (1.6 kgs) in the controlled community.

Furthermore, except for almonds, beans, avocados, and oils, most items in this diet are poor in calories. Consequently, even though you consume a significant amount of permitted items, it is impossible that this will result in calorie imbalance and contribute to weight gain.

Nevertheless, quite-low-calorie diets will typically not be managed in the long run. When they restore a regular eating schedule, most individuals who adopt these diets recover weight. Since amounts and portions are not defined by this diet, it is impossible to tell if it would supply sufficient calories for effective weight loss.

When adopting the diet or Sebi's menu, weight loss is expected to experience since the Sebi's diet is comprised of raw vegetables, fruits, wheat, nuts, and legumes.

It removes waste, sugar, poultry, and packaged foods, meaning you'll lose weight naturally. Dr. Sebi's diet works like a cleanser food and reaps several rewards, like your body praising you. It is also necessary, regularly, to drink a lot of water. This facilitates the separation from the body of the dangerous components. When this is the aim, it will help you achieve positive results during your journey towards weight loss.

One should consume about 1 gallon of pure water every day, according to Sebi. Do not drink tap water: always ensure that water you drink is 100% pure and clean.

3.8. How to reduce stress and increase cardiac function

Are you familiar with anxiety issues that impact over 18 percent of Americans? About 40 million citizens! This is more than 40 million! The proportion of youth is up to 25 percent. More than 284 million people around the world are impacted. Try to learn the ways through which we can take care of yourself and your health.

Stress and anxiety may contribute to a variety of health complications and mental health disorders. To avoid escalation, side effects and long-term effects, it's also necessary to treat anxiety as it arises. Although western healthcare practices rely on psychiatric care and medical intervention; several simple and easy methods prevent the risks related to anxiety and stress that can easily be adapted to overcome the issues.

Consequences of anxiety and stress and how to avoid:

The long-term impacts of anxiety may be severe; hence anxiety must be treated early and regularly so that serious harmful effects can be avoided and minimized. To stop the risks of fear and fatigue, adopt these basic tips:

1) Have some time for yourself because it is necessary. Life in modern society is too busy that we must calm down and relax occasionally. It is important to take some time to rest and get away from work to cope with chronic stress or anxiety. When the day ends, take some rest and enjoy a sample of Dr. Sebi's Tension Reliever Herbal tea, and spend some time with those you love most.

2) Manage time for those things which bring leisure to your life. Situations in which you do the only job, and no play must be avoided! Give yourself time for stuff you like. Do something that would help you feel comfortable every day so that the tension is eased. It doesn't mean to have tones of time — even fifteen to twenty minutes are enough.

3) One of the easiest methods of relaxing the body and mind is to do some exercise daily. This doesn't mean to be a strenuous activity, so it will enormously boost the mood by enjoying a walk after having your meals or resting before bed.

4) Stress can manage to take a toll on your normal defenses of the body. But having right diet can provide relaxation when consuming the right nutrients. Often the burden of everyday life is natural to feel wrung out. Sadly, we prefer to search for fast food, but do you know high-calorie or sugary snacks just trick us into believing that we feel stronger. Eating nutritious food will potentially give a serious stress reduction and make it a deliberate decision. Follow the Dietary Guide of Sebi and hydrate yourself properly to ensure that you have the right resources for your body to handle everything that comes to your way!

5) Breathing is considered a natural corporal feature and is taken for granted by most people. Stress, however, may cause individuals to slip into a dangerous pattern of breathing and fear. Generally, nervous people take quick, fast breaths at a rising pace. Although this is an indication of fear, it is, in reality, still a source that reinforces the sense of anxiety more. Anxiety contributes to shallow respiration, which contributes to further anxiety, contributing to shallower respiration, etc. As you can expect, everybody believes that building healthy breathing patterns is important and mentioned below are

some of the major health advantages of deep breathing techniques:

- Decreases your heart rate

- Control blood pressure

- Decrease build-up of lactic acid

- Core muscle stability is improved

- Decreases adverse effects of cortisol

- Immune system is boosted

- Volume of oxygen is increased being received by body

- Energy metabolism is increased

- Soothing effect on the brain

- Healing capabilities are improved

- Impacts positively on memory

- Improves capabilities for intense exercise.

- Electrical patterns are more organized in the brain

- Honor your heart just as nature demands

On average, a normal heart beats up to 42 million times during a year, pumping blood and creating an electromagnetic field that is detectable from 10 feet away. Unfortunately, the major cause of mortality in the US is heart disease; almost half of adults have cardiovascular complaints. But, remember, the heart is not just a pump, it is associated to love as well. So, think how much your heart is healthy?

Pressure built-up

Heart failure is triggered by congestion in the circulatory system. Blood arteries lose their resilience and cannot improve the heart's beating operation with their actual elasticity. Sugars and fats that are unsafe render them stiff and limit flow.

Blood pressure is increased by rigidity, causing the heart to work faster to force blood into the tissues. In this closed structure, mucus causes more pressure, putting more stress on the heart during pumping and lungs. Imagine pumping to dense pipe glue instead of liquid around the heating system. There's something about to blast!

Re-Engineering the Heart's Health

Before Sebi took decisive steps to resolve his health issues, he was really poor. He started consuming his native food and developed diabetes, hypertension, impotence, schizophrenia, and hysteria. It was the influence of diet and herbs that spared his life because medical technology did not save him. "The herbs are working for me," said Dr. Sebi, "and I realize I'm satisfied at 82."

Eating any food out of line with the cell predisposition induces illness. Impotence is an early warning indicator that the supply of blood is compromised. Luckily, enriching your body with blessings of nature restores wellness to every aspect of the body as well as mind.

Nourish your Heart

Addressing the dietary requirements of 'healthy' fats along with antioxidants found in nuts and seeds may be one of the easiest approaches to encourage cardiovascular health: consider consuming the following

- Reduces disease risk by using walnuts that contain alpha-linolenic acid.

- Brazil nuts have selenium that restores the equilibrium of fatty acids.

- Hemp seeds keep the blood vessels elastic and dilated.

- Sesame seed decreases cholesterol and eliminates inflammation.

Take diligent care of the cardiovascular function through diet, activity, and mind. A gentle, fun workout makes the core muscle healthy. Maintaining a balanced bodyweight and consuming food prevents the blood from circulating. Maintaining a good outlook promotes long-term well-being. Eat a nutritional diet given Sebi's Nutritional Guide. There are so many things you should do to hold the heart safe for a million more beats! Do you have heart disease following natural solutions.

Mother Nature offers all required essentials to restore dietary destruction and to clear up clogged arteries. When your heart wants extra help, Dr. Sebi's Green Food can softly put your heart muscle back into harmony. Cardiac-healthy herbs recommended by Dr. Sebi's Green Food dramatically improve the heart's health:

Bladderwrack eliminates the fatty deposits that clogged blood arteries.

Tila promotes relaxing, decreases inflammation and lowers blood pressure.

Nettle decreases blood glucose and blood pressure and reduces the chance of illness.

Nopal strengthens the nerves, decreases cholesterol and decreases blood sugar.

Dr. Sebi has also created herbal packets that contain the Lily of the Valley. It is a sweet-smelling plant and produces 40 different cardiac-glycosides that adjust fluid balance; boost contraction strength; restore heartbeat frequency, and overcome valve abnormalities.

Time to Change

Dr. Sebi has always been persistent in finding out the link between mental and physical healing. Dr. Sebi stated, "One of the elements that are so essential for this path to be recognized and understood is the LOVE, yet this was not the term itself. It's the electrical contact between you and any other guy or someone else besides you.

The electromagnetic fields of the hearts are built to bind us. It's beneficial to extend love and goodness. Translating passion into motion produces heartfelt echo and slavery. The basic act of smiling conveys optimistic feelings and awakens affection in the heart. Let's be heart-free, nutritiously free, and electromagnetically linked together.

Whatever you want to do, note that managing persistent stress and anxiety is just as vital to health as any other step you take.

Chapter 4. Dr. Sebi Soups Recipes

1. Dr. Sebi's" cleansing green soup

Serving: 4

Total Time: 1 hour

Ingredients:

- 3 if medium otherwise 2 large onions (yellow color), peeled and chopped them roughly.

- Zucchini 1, washed not peeled, and chopped roughly.

- Dandelion greens 1 bunch.

- Wild arugula1 bunch

- Vegetable broth homemade 4 cups (make it with approved vegetables only)

- Packed basil1/2 cup

- Packed dill1/2 cup

- key lime Juice of 1

- grapeseed oil 3 tbs

- sea salt 1/4 tbs

- avocado1/4

- Cayenne pepper, as per your taste

Directions:
To make this cleaning soup, begin to heat the grapeseed oil in

a wide pot on medium-high heat. Add the onion and then cook for 5 mins, stirring regularly, until translucent.

Add the dandelion greens, the zucchini and the wild arugula and simmer for another 5 minutes. Put in vegetable stock (homemade) and wait for a boil, decrease heat and let it cook, cover, for 15-20 minutes. Let it cool, with lid off, for 15 minutes.

If required, combine batches of basil, dill, avocado, lime, sea salt, juice and cayenne pepper, till very smooth. Serve and change the seasonings. Decorate with some new herbs.

If you prepare Dr. Sebi's Cleansing Green Soup, you are requested to please take a photo and share with the world on Sebi 's Official page of Facebook. We love if you share your experience with us.

2. Bell Pepper and Roasted Tomato Soup

Serving: 2

Total Time: 50 Minutes

Ingredients:

- Ripe Roma tomatoes 4

- red bell peppers 3

- fresh sprigs thyme 3

- Vegetable broth homemade 1/4 cup (make it with approved vegetables only)

- sea salt 100% pure according to your taste and some sesame oil

Directions:

Preheat your oven at 375 degrees F. Chop the peppers in quarter then cut the cores. Slice the tomatoes and put the bell peppers onto rimmed baking dish. Drizzle completely with the sesame oil and dust with sea salt. Spread the thyme all over the vegetables. Roast for about 35-40 minutes in a heated oven. Move everything into a blender or a food processor. Include the heated broth and the puree till it looks smooth, add more broth if required to obtain the perfect consistency.

Apply salt as per your taste. Pour in the bowls and serve.

3. Chickpea Soup

Serving: 4

Total Time: 30 minutes

Ingredients:

- Chickpeas 2 cups

- Zucchini 1 small size

- Bell pepper1

- Small onion1

- Water as required

- Seasoning with own choice

Directions:

Place all things in a pot and simmer over medium heat till vegetables are aldente. As soon as the soup gets ready and vegetables are cooked, take a multi-purpose blender and then blend them well. That's the best way to enjoy that. This is going to produce a soup for a couple of days.

4. Kale Soup

Serving: 2

Total Time: 30 minutes

Ingredients:

- onion chopped 1 medium size

- vegetable broth 5 cups

- chayote, diced 1 medium size

- squash, diced 2 cups

- kale 3 cups, rinsed, removed stems and fine chopped

- dried thyme 2 tbs

- dried sage two tbs

- pepper and salt as per taste

Directions:

Chop the onions and let them stay for 5 minutes. Warm one tabs of the broth in a medium pot. Saute the onion in the broth on medium heat, constantly stirring for 5 minutes. Add the broth and the chayote and bring to a boil. After heating, decrease the heat and proceed to cook for another five min. Add squash and simmer for around 15 min until soft. Add kale and remaining ingredients and simmer for another 5 mins. You want to cook longer for more taste and richness, then you may have to add a little more broth.

5. Alkaline Electric Soup

Serving:4

Total Time: 1.5 Hour

Ingredients:

- Approved Pasta/ Kamut Pasta 1-2 cups

- Quinoa Optional, 1/2 cup

- (cooked) Garbanzo Beans* 1/2 lb.

- Mushrooms, chopped 2 cups

- chopped Zucchini Squash 1

- chopped, Butternut Squash, 2 cups

- Green Peppers chopped, 1/2 cup

- Red Peppers chopped 1/2 cup

- chopped Red Onion small size, 1

- diced Roma Tomatoes, 2

- Spring Water 1/2 Gallon (adjust as required)

- Dill 1 tbs

- Red Cayenne Pepper 1 tbs

- Grapeseed Oil 1 tbs

- Oregano 1 tbs

- Basil 1 tbs

- Sea Salt 1 tbs

Directions:

Soak garbanzo beans in water overnight and boil them just before adding them to the Native Stew.

Pour spring water into a big pot and set the flame on medium heat.

Chop off all the herbs. Add the ingredients with seasonings to the pot and boil for around 1 hour. Stir the mixture every 15 minutes. Freeze the remaining stew for another day!

6. Greens Soup

Serving: 2

Total Time: 1 Hour

Ingredients:

- leafy greens 2 cups
- zucchini 1 small
- bell pepper 1
- onion 1 small
- Water as required
- Seasoning as per choice

Directions:

Put all ingredients in a pot and then cook over medium heat til the vegetables get semi-hard. Switch off the burner, let it cool and mix well togethe

Chapter 5. Dr. Sebi Salads

7. Cucumber Salad (Asian Style)

Serving: 1

Total time: 5 mins.

Ingredients:

- Key lime juice three tbs.

- Sesame oil 1 tbs.

- Date sugar 1/2 tsp.

- Sea salt 1/4 tsp.

- Ginger 1 tbs., in grated form

- Sesame seeds 1 tbs.

- Seaweed 1 tbs., in powdered granulated form

Direction:

To cook the Asian Cucumber Salad, simply pour it all together and enjoy it!

8. Basic Electric Chickpea or Bengal Gram Salad ("Tuna" Salad)

Serving: 2-4 **Total Time**: 1 hour 15 mins.

Ingredients

- Chickpeas 2 cups, properly cooked

- Basic Electric Hemp Seed Mayo 2/3 cup

- Red Onions 1/4 cup, chopped

- Green Peppers 1/8 cup, cubed

- Dulse Granules 1 tbsp. or Nori Sheet 1/2

- Onion Powder 2 tsp.

- Dill 1 tsp.

- Sea Salt 1/4 tsp.

- Masher

Dimensions:

Take chickpeas and add into the bowl and grind until the optimal texture has been achieved. If a sheet of Nori is used, split into tiny pieces and mix with the chickpeas. Mix the remaining

ingredients to the bowl and blend well. Keep it in refrigerator to cool for about 30 – 60 minutes before eating. Enjoy the Alkaline Electric Chickpea "Tuna" Salad!

9. Electric Pasta Salad (Alkaline)

Serving: 5-7

Total Time: 30 mins.

Ingredients

- Spelt Pasta/Basic Homemade Pasta 4 cups, cooked

- Bell Peppers 1 cup, either Red, Yellow or Green, cubed

- Zucchini/Summer Squash 1 cup, chopped

- Onions 1/2 cup, chopped

- Cherry Tomatoes 1/2 cup, cut them in two halves

- Black Olives 1/4 cup

- Alkaline "Garlic" Sauce 3/4 to 1 cup

Directions

Toss all the ingredients in a wide bowl once well combined and enjoy the Electric Pasta Salad (alkaline).

10. Quinoa Zucchini Salad

Serving: 12-14 slices

Total time: 50 mins.

Ingredients:

- Oregano 1 tsp.

- Spring Onion 2, finely sliced

- Olive Oil 3 tbsp.

- Zucchini 2, must be large & chopped

- Grapeseed Oil 2 tbsp.

- Key Lime Juice 1

- Chickpeas 15 oz. can

- Onion Powder 1 tsp.

- Quinoa 5 cup, properly cooked

Directions

First of all, take a tablespoon of oil into a large frying pan over medium flame. After this, now mix it in the slices of zucchini and simmer for three to four minutes or before tendering. Next is spooning in oregano and pour the residual oil into the pan.

In the final step, add cooked zucchini with the rest of the ingredients to a large bowl. Now toss well. It's ready to enjoy.

11.   Chickpeas (Bengali Gram) Salad

Serving: 3

Total times: 10 mins.

Ingredients:

- Chickpeas (Bengali gram) 1 ½ cups, drained & washed

- Red Onion ½ cup, cubed

- Cilantro ¼ cup, fresh one & well chopped

- Avocado 1 cup

- Sea Salt as per taste

Directions

First, put the chickpeas (Bengali gram) in a wide bowl then mash it with the masher. After doing this mash, the avocado now and then mixes it properly. In this mixture, add lemon juice and blend properly. Then whisk with the lime juice, blend and mix with the cilantro. Stir it again. Then, a spoon of salt. Whisk it again.

Serve and enjoy yourself.

12. Cucumber Mushroom Salad

Serving: 2.

Total time: 15 mins.

Ingredients:

- Olive Oil 1 tsp.

- Mushrooms 5, cut into two halves

- Key Lime Juice ½ of 1

- Olives 10

- Cherry Tomatoes 6, cut into two halves

- Sea Salt, as desired

- Lettuce leaves 6, rinsed

- Cucumber ½ of 1, sliced

Directions

Put the lettuce leaves, onions, mushrooms, olives, and cucumber in a wide mixing bowl to create this simple, balanced salad. After this, spill a spoon of olive oil along with the key lime juice on the salad. Toss it well. In the last, pour the sea salt on it. Toss the mixture well. Now enjoy yourself.

13.   Fruit Salad (Citrus)

Serving: 4

Total time: 50 mins.

Ingredients:

- Grapes 8 oz., seeded one

- Key Lime 1, should be quartered

- Medjool Dates 8, cut into two halves

- Kiwi 2, sliced

- Seville Oranges 4, skinned & sliced

Directions:

First, position all the ingredients required to produce the salad, excluding lime, in a wide mixing bowl. After this, squeeze the lime and pour it all over the salad, then toss properly. Serve, enjoy and love yourself.

14. Mashed Squash Salad

Serving: 6

Total time: 10 mins.

Ingredients:

- Allspice 1 tsp.

- Blue Agave ¼ cup, natural

- Squash 2, skinned & cubed

- Sea Salt 1/8 tsp.

- Date Sugar ¼ cup

- Hemp Milk ¼ cup

Directions

To start with, put the squash chunks and the water in a sauce-pan over medium flame. Boil the mixture and simmer for twenty minutes or when the squash is soft. When soft, clear the water then mash the squash. After this, add a spoon of date sugar, organic milk, allspice, sea salt and agave. Mix it well. Serve yourself and love it.

15. Watercress Salad

Serving: 2

Total time: 15 mins.

Ingredients:

- 1/8 tsp. Pure Sea Salt
- 4 cups Watercress, torn
- 2 tbsp. Olive Oil
- 1 Avocado, pitted, halved and sliced
- 2 tsp. Agave Syrup
- Cayenne Powder, as needed
- 2 Red Onions, sliced thinly
- 1 Seville Orange, peeled & cubed
- 2 tbsp. Key Lime Juice

Directions

First, take a mixing bowl, add orange, avocado, onion, and watercress. Now take another mixing bowl and add olive oil, the cayenne powder, key lime juice, agave syrup and the sea salt. Mix them well. Now, pour the olive oil dressing on the salad then toss it well. Serve the nutritious salad, enjoy and love it thoroughly.

Chapter 6: Dr. Sebi's Main Courses

16. Sautéed Greens

Serving: 8-10

Total Time: 15 minutes

Ingredients:

- Turnip Green, three bunches

- Pure Sea Salt, 3 tbsp.

- Onions 2 cups, chopped

- Cayenne Pepper, 1 tsp.

- Olive Oil, 1 tbsp.

Directions:

To begin, in a medium skillet, Saute onion over medium heat. After frying, add greens and roast for 18-20 minutes. Finally, season the mixture with cayenne pepper and salt.

17. Veggie Quinoa

Serving: 6-8

Total Time: 15 minutes

Ingredients:

- Basil, 1 tsp. Quinoa cooked 4 cups.

- Oregano 1 tsp. Zucchini chopped 1 cup.

- Pure Sea Salt 2 tsp.Red Bell Pepper ¼ cup, chopped

- Onion ½ cup, diced

- Green Bell Pepper¼ cup, chopped

- Cayenne Pepper ½ tsp.

- Yellow Bell Pepper ¼ cup, chopped

- Tomato 1 Plum, chopped

- Spring Water ½ cup

- Onion Powder 1 tbsp.

- Grape-seed Oil 2 tbsp.

Directions:

Begin by adding oil in a wide pan over medium heat. Then stir vegetables and season with the mixture and cook it for five minutes or before tender. Now, dump in the water together with the quinoa. Give it a nice swirl and finish cooking for two more minutes. Serve it.

18. Teff Porridge

Serving: 2

Total Time: 20 minutes

Ingredients:

- Spring Water, 2 cups

- Teff Grain 5 cups

- Sea Salt as required

- Agave Syrup 2 tbsp.

Directions:

First, boil the water into a pot on medium-high heat, then, as soon as it begins, Boil, whisk in the teff, then add the salt. Cover pot with the lid and lower the heat. Now, boil it for 10-15 minutes or till cooked. Serve with the seasoning of agave syrup and blueberries and serve.

19. Apple Quinoa Porridge

Serving:4

Total Time: 20 minutes

Ingredients:

- Key Lime ½ of 1

- Quinoa 5 cup; Apple 1 grated

- Coconut Oil 1 tbsp; Ginger 1-inch

Directions:

Begin with cooking the quinoa using the given instructions set on the envelope. Add the apple for five minutes until cooked. Now, simmer for half a minute and then add in the zest of lemon. The juice of the lemon to it. Next, stir the coconut oil, and mix well. Finally, scatter the mixture in the serving bowls. Garnish with the ginger.

20. Alkaline Electric Zucchini Bacon

Serving: 2-4

Total Time: 2 hours

Ingredients:

- Zucchini 2-3
- Date Sugar 1/4 cup
- Spring Water 1/4 cup
- Agave 2 tbsp.
- Sea Salt Smoked 1 tbsp.
- Onion Powder 1 tbsp.
- Liquid Smoke 1 tsp.
- Cayenne Powder 1/2 tsp.
- Ginger Powder 1/2 tsp.
- Mandoline / Potato Peeler
- Paper Parchment
- Grapeseed Oil

Directions:

Add all the ingredients into the saucepan and steam over low heat, and wait till they dissolved. Chop the zucchini and use the potato peeler to create the strips. In a wide bowl, mix the zucchini with the saucepan's ingredients and marinate for 30 to 60 minutes. There is no need for more water since it will come from zucchini. Use parchment paper on to the baking sheet and cover slightly with grape-seed oil. Cover the sheet with marinated strips, and bake at 400 ° F for ten minutes. Flip zucchini strips, cook 3-4 minutes, then leave to cool. If you like any of the strips to be crispy, roast for few more minutes or fry in a finely oiled pan for 30 sec. Enjoy the Alkaline-Electric-Bacon of Zucchini.

21. Vegetable Omelet

Serving: 1

Total Time: 25 minutes

Ingredients:

- Oregano ¼ tsp.

- Flour (Garbanzo Beans) ¼ cup

- Chopped Mushrooms ¼ cup

- Chopped Roma Tomato, ¼ cup

- Diced Green Pepper, ¼ cup

- Chopped Onion ¼ cup,

- Sea Salt 100% Pure ¼ tsp.

- Grapeseed Oil 1 tbsp.

- Onion Powder ¼ tsp

- Spring Water 1/3 cup

- Basil, sweet ¼ tsp.

- Cayenne Powder ¼ tsp.

Directions:

Start by putting garbanzo bean flour, include water and add seasoning in a wide mixing bowl. Whisk the combination properly, so it is properly blended. Heat oil in a large skillet on medium-high heat. When the oil is warmed, mix in a spoonful of all vegetables and the tomatoes. Sautee it for 2-3 minutes or before it becomes slightly tender.

Now add the flour mixture over it and blend it properly. Cook the mixture for 4 minutes, then turn mixture side by side. Using a spatula, remove the omelet's sides and turn it gently to the elevated position such that all parts of the omelet can be lifted. Only get fried. Serve them warm, please.

22.   Macaroni & Cheese

Serving: 10

Total Time: 45 minutes

Ingredients:

- Grapeseed Oil 2 tsp.

- Alkaline Pasta 12 oz.

- Juice 1 of ½ Key Lime

- Onion Powder 2 tsp.

- Garbanzo Flour ¼ cup

- Sea Salt 1 tsp.

- Spring Water 1 cup

- Raw Brazil Nuts 1 cup, overnight soaked

- Hempseed Milk 1 cup

- Achiote, grounded ½ tsp.

Directions:

Cook the pasta first according to the directions on the packet. Then, heat the oven to 350 F. Place the cooked pasta and drizzle oil over it into a baking dish. In a high-speed mixer, put all remaining ingredients and mix until the sauce gets creamy for 2 min or until ticked. Stir the cooked pasta with the sauce and chop it properly. Bake pasta for 20-30 minutes.

23. Mango Papaya Seed Dressing

Serving: 2

Total time: 3 mins.

- Ingredients
- Chopped Mango, 1 cup
- Grapeseed Oil 1/4 cup
- Lime Juice 2 tbsp.
- Ground Papaya Seed 1 tsp.
- Agave 1 tsp.
- Basil 1 tsp.
- Onion Powder 1 tsp.
- Sea Salt 1/4 tsp.

Directions:

Blend the ingredients inside blender and blend them for about a minute, it is now ready to serve.

24. Cucumber Dill Dressing

Serving: 2

Total time: 3 mins.

Ingredients:

- Chopped Plum Tomatoes, 2

- Sesame Seeds2 tbsp.

- Minced Onion, 1 tbsp.

- Agave 1 tbsp.

- Lime Juice 1 tbsp.

- Minced Ginger, 1 tsp.

Directions:

Start by blending all the ingredients in a blender and blend them for about 1&half minute, it is now ready to serve.

25. Alkaline Electric Mushroom & Onion Gravy

Serving: 3 **Total time**: 13 mins.

Ingredients:

- Spring Water 2-3 cups Mushrooms 1/2 cup

- Onions 1/2 Cup

- Garbanzo bean flour 3 tbs.

- Grapeseed Oil 2 tbs.

- Sea Salt 1 tsp.

- Onion Powder 1 tsp.

- Oregano 1/2 tsp.

- Thyme 1/2 tsp.

- Cayenne 1/4 tsp.

Directions:

Stir in skillet with grapeseed oil for about 2 minutes and Saute mushroos & onions with all spices and seasonings, bar cayenne. Add about 2 cups spring water. Then add cayenne powder and cook for five minutes. Mix it all up and get it to a boil. Proceed to cook to simmer, if necessary you can add remaining water. Enjoy your Alkaline Mushroom & Onion Gravy or your favorite meal with Kamut.

Chapter 7: Dr. Sebi's Dessert

26. Whipped Cream

Serving: 1

Total time: 15 mins.

Ingredients:

- Aquafaba 1 cup

- Agave Syrup ¼ cup

Directions

First, take the agave syrup and aquafaba in a small-medium size bowl and then mix them. Whisk the paste with a hand blender for about 10 to 15 minutes just until the cream becomes smooth.

27.   Blackberry Jam

Serving: 1

Total time: 15 mins.

Ingredients:

- Blackberries ¾ cup, fresh

- Sea Moss Gel ¼ cup

- Key Lime Juice 1 tbsp.

- Agave Syrup 3 tbsp.

Directions

Begin by putting the fresh blackberries in the medium-sized bowl over medium-high flame. Stirring constantly until you have a liquid mixture. When the berries have been soft, combine them in the processor until the batter is smooth and have no chunks.

Now, put the mixture back in the pot. Then take the sea moss gel with agave syrup, stir them with lime juice and add to the mixture. Next, boil the mixture until when it gets thickens. Stir it constantly. Take the pot out of the heat and let it cool down. Serve and love yourself

28. Dates Ball

Serving: makes 24 balls

Total time: 50 mins.

Ingredients:

- Walnuts ½ cup

- Sea Salt ½ tsp.

- Dates 1 cup, little bit pitted

- Agave Syrup ¼ cup

- Coconut Meat 1 cup

- Sesame Seeds ½ cup

Directions

Start by putting all the ingredients, excluding sesame seeds, in the processor and then blend them five times for about 20 seconds. Then switch the paste to a wide dish. Now, keep the balls out from the dish. Then dunk these balls in the sesame coats and then cover them deeply. Serve and love yourself.

29. Sweetened Chickpeas

Serving: 1

Total time: 50 mins.

Ingredients:

- Garbanzo Beans 15 oz., rinsed, drained & dry

- Agave Syrup 2 tbsp.

- Sea Salt ½ tsp.

- Olive Oil 1 tbsp.

Directions

Start with preheating the oven to 350 ft. Then add with the garbanzo beans, the sea salt, and the olive oil and agave syrup in a large mixing pan. Then mix well. Now move the paste into a baking tray lined with parchment paper, then distribute it thinly in a single sheet. Finally, bake for about 45 minutes, or when become crispy

30. Raisin Cookies

Servings: 2 **Total Time:** 45 Minutes

Ingredients:

- Applesauce 2/3 cup

- Raisins 1 cup

- Spelt Flour 1 ½ cup

- Pure Sea Salt ½ tsp.

- rolled Spelt flakes, 1 ½ cup

- Grapeseed Oil 1/3 cup

- Spring Water 2 tbsp.

- Dates pitted 1 ½ cup

- Agave 1/3 cup

Direction

To make these tasty cookies, all you need is to mix the spelled first. Add sea salt with dates into a food processor. Next, move the wheat mixture into a large bowl and then add the flour mixture. Add the spelled flakes. After that, blend all the remaining items and add them to the mixture. Have a good mix till you get a dough. Now, create the balls of dough and place them on a parchment baker's sheet. Make the balls flatten with a fork. Finally, bake them at 350 F about 20 minutes.

31.   Banana Walnut Ice Cream

Servings: 4

Total Time: 15 Minutes

Ingredients:

- Strawberries 1 cup

- chopped Avocado ½ of 1,

- Walnut Milk ¼ cup

- quartered Baby Bananas, 5

- Agave Syrup 1 tbsp.

Directions:

Start by adding all the ingredients into a high-speed blender you to make ice cream for 2 minutes. Add more walnut milk in case it is too thick. Then move the mixture to a broad freezer-safe tub. Then freeze it for 4 hours till it's set.

32. Walnut Date Nog

Servings: 2

Total Time: 10 Minutes

Ingredients:

- chopped Walnuts, ¼ cup

- Sea Salt ½ tsp.

- soaked Dates 4

- grounded Clove 1

- Hemp Seeds 4 tbsp.

- Dash of Anise

- Agave Syrup 2 tbsp.

- Spring Water 18 oz.

Directions:

Start by putting all the ingredients required to create the nog, except the clove and anise, inside a high-speed blender. Blend for about three minutes or till the mixture is smooth. Next, move the mixture into a medium-sized saucepan and heat. Serve with a slice of clove or anise. Enjoy it.

33. Strawberry Sorbet

Servings: 4

Total Time: 4 hours 10 minutes

Ingredients:

- Date Sugar ½ cup

- Strawberries 2 cups

- Spring Water 2 cups

- Spelt Flour 1 ½ tsp.

Directions:

Begin by combing date sugar, spelled flour, and spring water in a medium-sized pot. Next, heat the mixture over low heat and cook for 8 to 10 minutes or till thickened. After that, take off the pot from the heat and allow it to cool. Once cooled, puree the strawberries in a blender. Now, mix the strawberry puree to the flour mixture and give everything a good stir. Then, pour the mixture into a container and keep it in the freezer. Cut the frozen sorbet to pieces and place it in the blender or food processor. Blend until smooth and return the container to the refrigerator for a minimum of 4 hours.

Finally, serve the chilled strawberry sorbet.

34. Strawberry Ice Cream

Servings: 3 to 4

Total Time: 6 hours 10 Minutes

Ingredients:

- Hemp Milk ¼ cup
- frozen strawberries, 1 cup
- Agave Syrup 1 tbsp.
- frozen Baby Bananas, 5
- ripe Avocado, ½ of 1

Directions:

Place all ingredients necessary to make this ice cream into a high-speed blender. Mix them for 2-3 minutes or till the mixture is smooth. Check for sugar and, if appropriate, insert more agave syrup. Finally, move to the freezer-friendly jar and freeze for 4-6 hours

Chapter 8: Dr. Sebi's shakes

35. Detox Green Smoothie

Serving: 1

Total Time: 10 minutes

Ingredients:

- Greens Amaranth 2 cups

- Spring Water 2 cups

- Key Lime 1

- cored Apples, 2

- cubed Avocado, ¼ of 1

Directions:

- Put the greens, and avocado, with apple and key lime, high-speed blender adds appropriate amount of water. Blend the mixture for 1 to 1 ½ minutes, just before you get a rich and well-blended mixture. Serve and have fun.

36. Tomato Cucumber Smoothie

Serving: 1

Total Time: 10 minutes

Ingredients:

- Cucumber 1

- Agave Syrup3 tbsp.

- Plum Tomato 1

- Water 2 cups

Directions:

To create this tasty smoothie, combine all ingredients. Combine all ingredients for 2 to 3 minutes in a high-speed mixer till you get a rich and delicious smoothie.

37. **Peach Berry Smoothie**

Serving: 1

Total Time: 10 minutes

Ingredients:

- Sea Moss1 tbsp.

- Coconut Milk 1 cup

- Strawberries ½ cup

- Hemp Seeds 1 tbsp.

- quartered½ Peaches, cup

- Agave Syrup1 tbsp.

- Blueberries ½ cup

Directions:

Put bananas and agave syrup in a blender, add sea moss, hemp seed and coconut Milk, with blueberries and peaches in a high-speed blender. Blend the mixture for 1 minute or till you have a nice and luxurious smoothie. Transfer to the serving glass, drink instantly. Enjoy it!

Chapter 9: Dr. Sebi's Sauces

38. Salsa Verde

Serving: 2

Total Time: 10

Ingredients:

- Cilantro ¼ cup

- Onion Powder 1 tsp.

- Tomatillo, 1 lb. must be washed and skin removed.

- Pure Sea Salt 1 tsp.

- diced Onion ½ cup,

- Oregano 1 tsp.

Directions:

Start by putting the onions along with other ingredients to create this tasty dip. On Medium heat except for cilantro in a pan and fill it with water. Cook this mixture for 20 minutes, then stir from time to time. Then add the juice using a strainer. Next, transfer this whole mixture into a high-speed blender. Blend the mixture for about half a minute.

39. BBQ Sauce

Serving: 1 **Total Time**: 45 minutes

Ingredients:

- Cloves 1/8 tsp.

- Plum Tomatoes, 6

- Pure Sea Salt 2 tsp.

- chopped Onion, ¼ cup

- Onion Powder 2 tsp.

- Cayenne¼ tsp.

- Date Sugar ¼ cup

- Agave Syrup 2 tbsp.

Directions:

First, put all the ingredients required to make this sauce in a Mixer for high-speed. Mix them for 1-2 minutes or till a smooth paste is produced. Now pass the mixture into the tiny cup and drain date sugar from it. Cook on medium heat and mix regularly. Next, the heat should be low and allow the mixture to simmer for 15 minutes covered with a lid. Remember to stir frequently. Then mix in a blender until you get a smooth mixture using an immersion blender. Transfer the sauce again to the casserole and cook for another 10 minutes more. Let it cool down and then store.

40. Hot Sauce

Serving: 1

Total Time: 35 minutes

Ingredients:

- Sea Moss Powder 1 tbsp.

- Spring Water 1 ½ cups

- Onion Powder 2 tbsp.

- Key Lime Juice ½ cup

- Cayenne Pepper 2 tbsp.

- Plum Tomatoes 9

- Pure Sea Salt ½ tsp.

Directions:

Start with all ingredients to create the hot sauce. Mix and blend it in a high-speed blender for 3 minutes or before you obtain a smooth paste. Then heat this mixture over medium heat. Cook the mixture around 10-15 minutes, then let it cool. Store in a glass jar. Snacks and bread based on Doctor Sebi products.

Chapter 10: Training strategy

Getting Ready for Dr. Sebi Diet.

Since first beginning following Sebi's and telling friends and family regarding his plans, most of them seem to have reservations that one might not adjust to such a diet and lifestyle. But here for the 6th year, and its always going high.

Like other people, everybody I spoke to looked at things the wrong way – concentrating on the drawbacks of the food rather than possibilities. I guess the biggest explanation for this is that, for those living on fast food and pre-packaged garbage, much of the food in Sebi's list may sound a little foreign because there's a lot of stuff out there by using which you can create hearty meals.

My tips on people trying to follow a Sebi diet are simple. Below, I'm going to go through the key stuff I wish anyone had taught me when I first began doing this years ago. Anyways if you're still not sure what this diet means to take a peek at my webpage. I'm providing a rundown, along with some advantages.

Be armed physically and psychologically to fully adjust to Serbian's eating style. You may have to begin by making certain adjustments to your overall lifestyle. You're likely to discover that this allows people to be in the correct state of mind and mental condition.

Eating is part of life, and the kinds of foods or drugs we eat daily shape solid behaviors that will last for a lifetime if we left them unchecked.

These patterns may be incredibly difficult to overcome or alter. The power of the culture and people nearest to us may also be a hindrance.

That's why, before you rush into this diet style, you can take more time dreaming about improving your food don't pledge something then just struggle because of lack of planning, family problems, or something, then break something pledge.

Start consuming some of the water is important to cleanse your bodies, sustain balanced brain or body functions, with a variety of other benefits.

It recommends consuming up to 1 gallon of fresh spring water a day. Springwater is preferred since it is usually alkaline instead of tap water, rich in chlorine and other toxins.

Begin reading the ingredients labels. It's not going to be convenient for certain people to give-up those sweets or soft beverages. Hence, a perfect way to get started is to scan the food product labels. It's a great idea and an utter requirement to be mindful of what you're consuming and drinking. At first, if you don't eat based on the food chart, this knowledge may allow you to improve your behaviors as you advance.

Snacking in the best way. Snacking may be a compulsive activity, but it doesn't suggest it has to be a poor one. Most people enjoy snacks many times, but instead of finding a bag full of chips or a big chocolate bar, why not consider making your snacks mix of walnuts and raisins along with other dried fruits.

When you pass the line from packaged eating to cooking every day, the road to health rehabilitation and control gets even smoother. You can soon see the countless possibilities available and learn how you can take your beloved recipes and re-make them like accepted recipes to experience the same meals you've always had.

Begin eating Irish moss: Get associated with Irish sea-moss try producing a gel. This is one of your diet pillars because it's healthy and it's tasteless, so you can apply it to any of your favorite meals without really knowing it's there.

Introduce authorized foods from Dr. Sebi. When you're finished, print out the food list and select a couple of foods you know about, replacing whatever you can with products on in list from your current diet.

Empower yourself with some recipes authorized by Sebi.

I've already put together a compilation of easy to prepare Sebi's approved recipes. Now I recommend you take a couple of them and start replacing some of the traditional meals every week.

Conclusion

Dr. Sebi ties the connections between physical and mental disorders and nutrition. A skeletal human, anyone lacking in vitamins and nutrients, has a brain that breaks down, resulting in irrational thought and, eventually, dangerous behavior. If the body gets everything it wants, it's calm. Healing the intestines by eliminating contaminants is related to healing the brain. A toxin is removed from an alkaline diet devoid of acid-based foods. Happiness is affected if the organism is acidic. When the body is extremely acidic, instability, madness, discontent, and aggression occur.

CPSIA information can be obtained
at www.ICGtesting.com
Printed in the USA
LVHW011636230621
690870LV00013BB/756

9 781801 922654